Contents

mechanical methods, without the prior written permission of the publisher, except in the case of brief quotations embodied in critical reviews and certain other noncommercial uses permitted by copyright law.

Abstract

"Pawsitively Healthy Smiles: The Comprehensive Guide to Canine Dental Care" serves as an invaluable resource for dog owners, offering a holistic exploration of the significance of dental health in dogs. Beyond the pursuit of fresh breath, this guide emphasizes the profound impact of good oral hygiene on a dog's overall well-being, longevity, and quality of life.

The guide navigates through common oral conditions such as tooth resorption, fractured teeth, persistent deciduous teeth, and dental malocclusions, providing insights into recognition and prompt treatment. Essential dental care practices, including the gold standard of toothbrushing and alternative options like dental chews and sprays, are detailed with practical guidance for implementation.

Highlighting the necessity of professional veterinary cleanings, the guide outlines their role in complementing at-home care, detecting unnoticed oral problems, and ensuring a comprehensive cleaning process. The chapter on dealing with stained teeth delves into the importance of regular toothbrushing, professional veterinary dental care, and maintaining a bright and healthy smile for dogs.

In conclusion, the guide reinforces the importance of investing time and effort into a dog's dental care, summarizing key takeaways and providing a call to action for pet owners. With a focus on prevention, early intervention, and a comprehensive approach, "Pawsitively Healthy Smiles" aims to empower dog owners to prioritize their canine companions' oral health for a lifetime of optimal smiles and well-being.

Introduction

Welcome to "Pawsitively Healthy Smiles: The Comprehensive Guide to Canine Dental Care." As devoted dog owners, we understand the profound connection we share with our furry friends. Beyond the wagging tails and playful antics, the well-being of our dogs encompasses every aspect of their health, and dental care plays a pivotal role in ensuring their overall happiness and longevity.

This comprehensive guide embarks on a journey through the intricate world of canine dental health, transcending the conventional view of dental care merely as a means to achieve fresh breath. We delve into the significance of good oral hygiene, exploring its direct link to a dog's holistic well-being. From the prevention of common oral conditions to essential dental care practices, we aim to equip dog owners with the knowledge and tools needed to become proactive stewards of their pets' oral health.

Throughout the guide, we'll unravel the mysteries of tooth resorption, fractured teeth, persistent deciduous teeth, and dental malocclusions, providing insights into recognizing and addressing these conditions promptly. We'll guide you through essential dental care practices, including the gold standard of toothbrushing, as well as alternative options for those who find brushing challenging.

Acknowledging the collaborative effort between dog owners and veterinary professionals, we underscore the importance of regular veterinary cleanings. These cleanings, complementing at-home care, become crucial in detecting unnoticed oral problems and ensuring a thorough and comprehensive approach to your dog's oral health.

Finally, we tackle the challenge of stained teeth, emphasizing the importance of regular toothbrushing, seeking professional veterinary dental care when needed, and maintaining a commitment to preventive measures. We believe that a healthy smile not only contributes to a dog's physical well-being but also enhances the joy they bring to our lives.

As you embark on this educational journey with "Pawsitively Healthy Smiles," may you discover the keys to unlocking a lifetime of optimal oral health for your beloved canine companions. After all, a healthy smile leads to a happy dog!

Chapter One

The Significance of Dental Health for Dogs

Beyond Fresh Breath

The importance of canine dental health extends far beyond the desire for fresh breath. While a minty-fresh odor from your dog's mouth is undoubtedly pleasant, it is merely a side effect of proper oral care. In reality, good dental health is intricately connected to your dog's overall well-being and longevity. Just as in humans, the mouth serves as a gateway to the body, and neglecting oral hygiene can lead to a cascade of health issues.

Dental problems in dogs can range from mild to severe, impacting not only the mouth but also various organs and systems. Poor oral hygiene can result in the accumulation of plaque, a biofilm of bacteria that adheres to the teeth. If left untreated, this can progress to tartar, which harbors more harmful bacteria and can cause inflammation of the gums (gingivitis). The consequences of untreated dental issues go beyond discomfort; they can lead to infections, compromised organ function, and a reduced quality of life for your canine companion.

Overall Well-being and Longevity

Maintaining your dog's dental health is a holistic approach to ensuring their overall well-being and promoting a longer, healthier life. Studies have shown that dogs with good oral hygiene tend to live longer than those with neglected dental care. This correlation is not coincidental; rather, it underscores the profound impact that oral health can have on the entire body.

Poor dental health in dogs has been linked to various systemic conditions, including heart disease, kidney disease, and diabetes. The connection lies in the circulation of bacteria and inflammatory substances from the mouth to other organs through the bloodstream. By preventing oral issues through regular dental care, you are not only preserving your dog's teeth and gums but also safeguarding their vital organs and systems.

Link to Systemic Health Problems

The intricate relationship between oral health and systemic well-being cannot be overstated. Bacteria originating from dental problems can enter the bloodstream, triggering inflammation and potentially affecting distant organs. In the case of the heart, this can contribute to the development of endocarditis, an inflammation of the heart's inner lining. Similarly, the kidneys may suffer from compromised function due to the systemic effects of oral bacteria.

Beyond infections, untreated dental conditions can also exacerbate pre-existing health issues in dogs. For instance, diabetic dogs may experience difficulty regulating blood sugar levels if oral infections are present. This interplay between dental health and systemic conditions emphasizes the need for a proactive approach to canine dental care, involving both at-home practices and regular professional cleanings.

In summary, recognizing the significance of dental health for dogs goes beyond the superficial concern of breath freshness. It involves understanding the profound impact that oral care has on your dog's overall well-being, longevity, and quality of life. As responsible pet owners, it is our duty to prioritize and actively engage in practices that ensure our furry friends enjoy optimal oral health throughout their lives.

Chapter Two

Common Oral Conditions in Dogs

Tooth Resorption

Tooth resorption is a relatively common dental issue in dogs, characterized by the gradual breakdown and loss of tooth structure. This process can be painful for your furry friend and is often associated with factors such as inflammation, genetics, and oral trauma. Identifying tooth resorption early is crucial, as advanced cases may necessitate tooth extraction to alleviate discomfort and prevent further complications.

Regular dental check-ups are essential for detecting signs of tooth resorption, such as changes in tooth color, sensitivity, or difficulty while eating. Dental X-rays are particularly valuable in identifying the extent of resorption below the gumline, guiding veterinarians in making informed treatment decisions.

Fractured Teeth

Dogs, especially those with a penchant for chewing hard objects or engaging in vigorous play, are susceptible to fractured teeth. Fractures can range from minor chips to more severe breaks that expose the pulp chamber, leading to pain and potential infections. Fractured teeth may not always be visually obvious, making regular dental examinations critical for early detection.

Prompt intervention is crucial when a fractured tooth is identified. Depending on the severity, treatment options may include bonding, crowns, or in severe cases, extraction. Ignoring fractured teeth can result in persistent pain, the spread of infection, and compromised oral function.

Persistent Deciduous Teeth

In some cases, a dog's baby teeth (deciduous teeth) may not fall out naturally, leading to the persistence of two sets of teeth in the mouth. This can cause misalignments and impede proper jaw development. Timely identification and extraction of retained deciduous teeth are necessary to prevent complications such as malocclusions and overcrowding.

Regular monitoring of your puppy's dental development and consulting with your veterinarian can aid in identifying and addressing issues related to persistent deciduous teeth. Early intervention ensures that your dog's adult teeth can erupt properly, setting the foundation for a healthy and well-aligned dentition.

Dental Malocclusions

Dental malocclusions refer to misalignments of the teeth and jaws, impacting both the appearance and functionality of your dog's bite.

These conditions can be congenital or develop over time, affecting various breeds differently. Malocclusions may lead to oral discomfort, difficulty eating, and an increased risk of dental issues.

Identifying dental malocclusions often involves a comprehensive dental examination and, in some cases, dental X-rays to assess the alignment of the teeth below the gumline. Treatment options may include orthodontic devices, tooth extractions, or other corrective measures, depending on the nature and severity of the malocclusion.

Prompt Recognition and Treatment

Recognizing and addressing common oral conditions in dogs require a proactive approach to dental care. Regular at-home dental examinations, coupled with professional veterinary check-ups, form a comprehensive strategy for early detection. Understanding the signs and symptoms associated with tooth resorption, fractured teeth, persistent deciduous teeth, and dental malocclusions empowers dog owners to seek timely veterinary intervention, thereby ensuring their canine companions enjoy optimal oral health and comfort.

In the next section, we will explore essential dental care practices that can be implemented at home to prevent these common oral conditions and promote a lifelong journey of healthy smiles

for your furry friend.

Chapter Three

Essential Dental Care Practices

Brushing Your Dog's Teeth

Brushing your dog's teeth is the gold standard of canine dental care. It serves as a proactive measure to remove plaque, prevent bad breath, decay, and gum disease. To embark on a successful toothbrushing routine, consider the following steps:

Choosing the Right Tools

Selecting a suitable dog toothbrush and toothpaste is fundamental. Dog-specific toothbrushes with soft bristles and flavored toothpaste formulated for canines make the experience more enjoyable. Introduce these tools gradually, allowing your dog to acclimate to the textures and tastes.

Gradual Introduction to Toothbrushing

Familiarize your dog with the sensation of having their teeth touched. Begin by gently rubbing their gums with your finger, then introduce the toothbrush in a non-threatening manner. Progress slowly, ensuring your dog is comfortable at each stage.

Positive Reinforcement

Make the toothbrushing experience positive by offering praise and rewards. Use treats or verbal affirmations to create a connection between toothbrushing and positive outcomes. Consistency is key to establishing a routine that your dog associates with care and affection.

Regular toothbrushing, ideally a few times per week, helps maintain your dog's oral health, preventing the buildup of plaque and reducing the risk of common dental issues.

Alternative Dental Care Options

If toothbrushing proves challenging for your dog, alternative dental care options offer effective alternatives to maintain their oral health:

Dental Chews

Dental chews provide a tasty treat that also aids in cleaning your dog's teeth. The chewing action helps reduce plaque and tartar buildup. Choose chews designed to promote dental health, and ensure they are an appropriate size for your dog's breed and size.

Dental Sprays

Dental sprays offer a convenient way to freshen your dog's breath and provide additional oral care between brushings. These sprays often contain antibacterial agents that help combat the growth of harmful bacteria in the mouth.

Chew Toys

Satisfy your dog's natural chewing instincts with appropriate chew toys. Certain toys are designed to promote dental health by reducing plaque and tartar. Look for options with textures that help clean teeth as your dog chews.

By incorporating these alternative options into your dog's routine, you can contribute to their oral hygiene even if traditional toothbrushing is not feasible.

In the following section, we will delve into the importance of professional veterinary cleanings as a complementary measure to at-home dental care, ensuring a comprehensive approach to your dog's oral health.

Chapter Four

Professional Dental Cleanings

The Importance of Regular Veterinary Cleanings

While at-home dental care practices are crucial for maintaining your dog's oral health, professional cleanings by a veterinarian play a pivotal role in comprehensive dental care. Here's why regular veterinary cleanings are essential:

Complementing At-Home Care

Professional dental cleanings serve as a complement to your at-home dental care efforts. Despite your best intentions and practices, certain areas of your dog's mouth may be challenging to reach or clean thoroughly. Veterinary cleanings ensure a comprehensive removal of plaque and tartar, particularly in areas that are difficult to access during routine home care.

Detecting Unnoticed Oral Problems

Veterinarians are trained to identify and address oral problems that may go unnoticed by pet owners. During a professional cleaning, the veterinarian can identify issues such as early signs of periodontal disease, infections, or abnormalities that may require further investigation or treatment.

Scaling, Polishing, and Radiographs

Professional cleanings involve a thorough process that goes beyond what can be achieved at home. This includes scaling to remove tartar and plaque both above and below the gumline, polishing to smooth the tooth surfaces and discourage plaque buildup, and the use of dental radiographs to assess the health of the teeth and supporting structures.

Frequency of Veterinary Cleanings

The frequency of professional dental cleanings may vary based on factors such as your dog's age, breed, and overall dental health. In general, annual veterinary cleanings are recommended, but certain breeds or dogs with specific oral health concerns may require more frequent cleanings.

What to Expect During a Veterinary Cleaning

Understanding what occurs during a veterinary cleaning can help alleviate any concerns and reinforce the importance of this aspect of canine dental care:

General Anesthesia for Stress-Free Experience

To ensure a stress-free and safe experience, your dog will be placed under general anesthesia during the veterinary cleaning. This not only allows for a more thorough examination and cleaning but also ensures your dog remains calm and comfortable throughout the procedure.

Thorough Cleaning Below the Gumline

The veterinarian will carefully clean your dog's teeth, paying special attention to the areas below the gumline where tartar and plaque can accumulate. This is a critical step in preventing and addressing periodontal disease, a common and often painful condition in dogs.

Comprehensive Oral Examination

In addition to cleaning, the veterinarian will conduct a comprehensive oral examination. This may involve evaluating the gums, teeth, tongue, and other oral structures. Any abnormalities or issues discovered during this examination will be addressed accordingly.

Dental Radiographs and Additional Treatments

Dental radiographs (X-rays) may be taken to assess the health of the tooth roots and surrounding structures. If any dental issues are identified, such as cavities, fractures, or abscesses, appropriate treatments, such as fillings or extractions, will be performed.

Regular veterinary cleanings, combined with consistent at-home dental care practices, contribute significantly to maintaining your dog's oral health and preventing serious dental problems.

In the next section, we will explore the importance of regular toothbrushing in preventing stained teeth and maintaining a bright and healthy smile for your furry friend.

Chapter Five

Dealing with Stained Teeth

Importance of Regular Toothbrushing

Prevention is key when it comes to stained teeth in dogs. Regular toothbrushing serves as a fundamental practice to maintain oral health and prevent the formation of unsightly stains. Here's why incorporating toothbrushing into your dog's routine is crucial:

Plaque and Stain Prevention

Plaque, a biofilm of bacteria, is a precursor to both dental issues and teeth staining. Regular toothbrushing helps remove plaque, reducing the likelihood of stains forming on your dog's teeth. By brushing your dog's teeth consistently, you contribute to the prevention of both oral health problems and cosmetic concerns.

Removal of Surface Stains

Surface stains caused by factors like diet, age, and certain medications can often be mitigated through regular toothbrushing. The mechanical action of brushing helps remove superficial discoloration, keeping your dog's teeth looking cleaner and brighter.

Maintaining Fresh Breath

Beyond aesthetics, regular toothbrushing contributes to fresher breath by eliminating the bacteria responsible for bad odors. A clean and healthy mouth translates to a more pleasant experience for both you and your canine companion.

Establishing a Positive Routine

Introducing toothbrushing as a positive and routine aspect of your dog's care from an early age creates a lifelong habit. Dogs who are accustomed to regular toothbrushing are more cooperative, making the process smoother for both pet owners and their furry friends.

Professional Veterinary Dental Care

If your dog's teeth are severely stained, or if you encounter challenges in maintaining their oral health, seeking professional veterinary dental care is essential:

Scaling Away Tartar and Polishing

A veterinary dentist can perform a professional dental cleaning to address stubborn tartar and stains. This involves scaling to remove accumulated plaque and tartar and polishing to restore a smoother and cleaner tooth surface.

Resuming Toothbrushing Post-Professional Cleaning

While professional veterinary dental care can significantly improve the appearance of stained teeth, it's crucial to resume regular toothbrushing immediately afterward. Consistent at-home dental care is essential for maintaining the benefits of the professional cleaning and preventing future stains and oral health issues.

In conclusion, addressing stained teeth in dogs involves a proactive approach that combines regular toothbrushing with professional veterinary dental care when needed. By prioritizing your dog's oral health, you not only enhance their appearance but also contribute to their overall well-being and longevity.

The journey to a pawsitively healthy smile for your furry friend involves consistent dental care practices, both at home and with the guidance of your veterinarian. By implementing the strategies outlined in this guide, you are taking significant steps towards ensuring your dog enjoys a lifetime of optimal oral health and a sparkling smile.

In the final section, we'll recap the key takeaways and reinforce the importance of investing time and effort into your dog's dental care.

Conclusion

Congratulations on reaching the end of "Pawsitively Healthy Smiles: The Comprehensive Guide to Canine Dental Care." Throughout this guide, we've explored the significance of dental health for dogs, common oral conditions, essential dental care practices, the importance of professional veterinary cleanings, and strategies for dealing with stained teeth.

Key Takeaways:

Beyond Fresh Breath

- Understand that dental health is integral to your dog's overall well-being and longevity.
- Poor oral hygiene can lead to painful conditions, infections, and systemic health problems.

Common Oral Conditions

- Recognize and address issues like tooth resorption, fractured teeth, persistent deciduous teeth, and dental malocclusions promptly.

Essential Dental Care Practices

- Embrace toothbrushing as the gold standard for dental care.

- Gradually introduce your dog to toothbrushing, use positive reinforcement, and make it a positive experience.

- Explore alternative options like dental chews, sprays, and chew toys.

Professional Veterinary Cleanings

- Acknowledge the necessity of regular cleanings by a veterinarian.

- Understand the comprehensive nature of veterinary cleanings, including scaling, polishing, and dental radiographs.

Dealing with Stained Teeth

- Prioritize regular toothbrushing to prevent stains and maintain a clean and bright smile.

- Seek professional veterinary dental care for severe stains, followed by consistent at-home care.

Conclusion and Call to Action

By prioritizing your dog's dental care, you are not only investing in their immediate comfort but also ensuring their long-term health and happiness. Regular toothbrushing, alternative dental care options, and professional veterinary cleanings collectively contribute to a comprehensive approach.

Remember

- Dental care should start early, from puppyhood.

- Different dog breeds may have specific dental needs.

- Always consult with your veterinarian for personalized dental care advice.

Invest the time and effort into your dog's dental care, and you'll be rewarded with a furry friend who not only has a healthy smile but also enjoys a higher quality of life. A healthy smile truly leads to a happy dog!

Thank you for embarking on this journey towards optimal canine oral health. May your dog's smiles always shine bright!